THE UNPLEASANT TRINITY:

How CRABS, SUGAR and OILS make us obese, unhealthy and Intoxicated and how to break free.

By
Jeffrey W. Aviles

Table of contents

Introduction

With regards to disease, what does 'main cause' really mean? What's more, what difference does it make? Laying out the underlying driver of an infection implies resolving WHY it has worked out. For what reason does THIS individual have THIS specific disease? What are the variables that drove doing it?

It makes a difference since it assists with recognizing basic brokenness that could be adding to your side effects and tending to these is a significant piece of further developing wellbeing. On the off chance that you take a gander at the branches of the tree above, you can see that there are various infections that an individual could endure. Furthermore, under, you can see an extensive variety of root causes. Of course, this is not a comprehensive rundown of illnesses, yet the point is to outline that numerous illnesses have a typical assortment of hidden brokenness (main cause).

As a matter of fact, there is a staggering measure of proof that connects our eating regimen, way of life, and climate with constant diseases.There are

outstanding advances in both treatment and counteraction of numerous intense medical conditions in ordinary medication, for example, for contaminations and sorts of injury. Be that as it may, in treating and forestalling persistent infection, regular medication has not been as viable.

As of now, when there is a conclusion of a persistent infection, it is generally circled back to a solution for a medication to deal with the side effects. Yet, side effect concealment doesn't manage the underlying driver and may bring about additional medical issues in the future.So, instead of zeroing in just on freeing the side effects from persistent sickness, which is in many cases simply a bandage or brief fix, it means quite a bit to take a gander at where the brokenness might begin. We ought to zero in on mediation informed by science to address the illness as its main causes. This assists with forestalling future ailment, alleviating

side effects, and switching the movement of the momentum sickness.

Sicknesses are often complicated and multifactorial with interconnected organic frameworks, which is the reason addressing underlying drivers to further develop well-being implies viewing every individual in general, as opposed to a little piece of that entirety. Taking a gander at the main driver of infection can frequently feel like criminal investigator work. I had two clients as of late who were both determined to have Hashimoto's sickness, were generally solid, and couldn't comprehend how they had fostered a thyroid problem. Even though the two of them had similar findings and were on similar prescriptions, the areas of brokenness were exceptional for every client.

One had numerous food awarenesses which should have been addressed and the other was routinely presented to poisons in her current circumstance. Addressing these main causes had a huge effect on their side effects. You should be an accomplice in your medical services when you have constant sickness. Check out the roots on the tree. Which

could you at any point address? Might you at any point get an additional hour of rest this evening, or take a walk as opposed to plunk down before the television? Now and again these little changes can add up to enormous well-being gains. Everyone is unique, which is the reason this approach should be customized. Work with me by assuming a functioning part in your excursion to further develop your well-being.

PART ONE

What you want to be familiar with your well-being.

Chapter 1:

Excessive Cholesterol

Excessive cholesterol is firmly connected with numerous other clinical issues. That implies it can lead to a few difficult issues to begin (like coronary course illness). Yet, it can likewise occur because of different illnesses, particularly ones that trigger irritation in your body (like lupus). Individuals with excessive cholesterol frequently foster hypertension too.

What is Excessive cholesterol Excessive cholesterol is the point at which you have a lot of cholesterol in your blood, which can expand the gamble of having a cardiovascular failure or stroke.It's likewise called hyperlipidemia or hypercholesterolemia. Your body needs an ideal extent of lipids to work. Assuming you have such a large number of lipids, your body can't utilize them all. The extra lipids start to foster in your arteries. They join with different substances in your blood to shape plaque (greasy deposits). This plaque probably won't lead to any issues for a long time, yet after some time, the plaque quietly gets increasingly big inside your arteries. To this end untreated excessive cholesterol is risky. Those additional lipids in your blood assist with making the plaque greater without you in any event, knowing it. The best way to realize you have excessive cholesterol is through a blood test. A blood test, called a lipid board, lets you know the number of lipids that are circling in your blood. What is viewed as excessive cholesterol depends upon your age, sex, and history of coronary illness.

Good cholesterol vs Bad cholesterol

There are a few sorts of lipids. The fundamental ones you've likely probably heard of are "Good cholesterol" and "Bad cholesterol." Good cholesterol is called high-thickness lipoprotein (HDL). Consider the "H" as"Helpful." Your HDLs convey cholesterol to your liver. Your liver keeps your cholesterol levels adjusted. It makes sufficient cholesterol to help your body's necessities and disposes of the rest. You should have an adequate number of HDLs to convey cholesterol to your liver. Assuming your HDLs are excessively low, you'll have a lot of cholesterol circling in your blood.

Bad cholesterol is called low-thickness lipoprotein (LDL). This is the guilty party that makes plaque structure in your arteries. Having such a large number of LDLs can prompt coronary illness over the long run.

When to have your cholesterol Examine

Excessive cholesterol can begin in youth or immaturity.That is the reason current rules recommend starting screenings during adolescence. **Kids and adolescents:** Have your cholesterol examine every 5 years intervals beginning at age nine. A youngster whose guardians have excessive cholesterol or a past filled with heart issues might start even sooner.

Individuals assigned male at birth (AMAB): Have your cholesterol examined every 5 years intervals until age 45. From age 45 to 65, get examine every one to two years. After age 65, get examined each year.

Individuals assigned female at birth(AFAB): Get examined every 5years until age 55. From age 55 to 65, get an examination every one to two years. After age 65, get examined each year. These are overall rules. Your medical care supplier will examine what's best for you. For instance, somebody in their 20s with excessive cholesterol numbers might require yearly tests for some time. Individuals with other coronary illness risk variables might require more regular tests, as well.

Source of Excessive Cholesterol

Way of life variables and hereditary qualities both play a part in causing excessive cholesterol. Way of life factors includes:

Smoking and tobacco use: Smoking brings down your "Good cholesterol" (HDL) and raises your "Bad cholesterol" (LDL).

Being under a ton of stress: Stress triggers hormonal changes that make your body produce cholesterol.

Drinking liquor: An excess of liquor in your body can raise your absolute cholesterol.

Not moving around enough: Actual work like oxygen-consuming activity further develops your cholesterol numbers. If you have a work area work or sit a great deal of your spare energy, your body won't create enough "great cholesterol."

Diet: A few food sources might raise or lower your cholesterol. Here and there medical care suppliers will suggest dietary changes or an encounter with a nutritionist to examine your eating regimen.

Signs of Excessive cholesterol

Excessive cholesterol causes no signs for most people. You could be a long-distance runner and have excessive cholesterol. You won't begin to feel any signs until the excessive cholesterol leads to different issues in your body. Excessive cholesterol raises your gamble of conditions like fringe supply route sickness, hypertension, and stroke. Excessive cholesterol is normal among individuals with diabetes.

How does excessive cholesterol influence my body

Over the long run, excessive cholesterol prompts plaque development inside your veins. This plaque development is called atherosclerosis. Individuals with atherosclerosis face a higher threat of a wide range of ailments. That is because your veins accomplish significant work all through your body. So when there's an issue in one of your veins, there's a ripple effect. You can consider your veins a perplexing organization of lines that keep blood moving through your body. Plaque resembles the gunk that obstructs your lines at home and slows down your shower channel. Plaque adheres to the internal walls of your veins and cutoff points to how much blood can stream through. When you have excessive cholesterol, you have plaque shaping inside your veins. The more you do without treatment, the greater the plaque gets. As the plaque gets greater, your veins become limited or obstructed. Like a mostly stopped-up channel, your veins might in any case work for quite a while. In any case, they won't fill in as productively as they should. High cholesterol raises your gamble of other ailments relying upon which veins are stopped.

Coronary artery disease(CAD).

Coronary Artery Disease (CAD) is additionally called coronary heart disease(CHD) or ischemic coronary illness. This is the very thing most people mean when they utilize the expression "coronary disease." CAD is the most well-known type of coronary disease in the U.S. furthermore, the main source of death. CAD occurs at the point when atherosclerosis influences your coronary veins. These are the veins that convey blood to your heart. At the point when your heart doesn't get sufficient blood, it gets more vulnerable and quits filling in as it ought to. CAD can prompt a coronary episode or heart failure. What many individuals don't know is that CAD can influence more youthful individuals. Truth be told, around 1 out of 5 individuals who pass on from CAD are under age 65. That is the reason it's vital to have your cholesterol examine beginning quite early on. Over the long haul, plaque can quietly develop in your coronary supply routes. Many individuals don't understand it's occurring until they get chest torment (angina) or one more indication of cardiovascular failure.

Carotid artery disease: When atherosclerosis influences your carotid artery, it's called carotid artery disease. Your carotid arteries convey blood to the huge, forward portion of your cerebrum. At the point when plaque limits these arteries, your mind can't get sufficient oxygen-rich blood. Carotid artery disease can prompt a transient ischemic assault (TIA or "scaled down stroke") or a stroke.

Peripheral artery disease (PAD)

When atherosclerosis influences the arteries in your legs or arms, it's called Peripheral artery disease (PAD) The arteries in your legs and arms are "peripheral" since they're away from your heart and the focal point of your body. PAD is more normal in your legs however can likewise occur in your arms. PAD is hazardous because it frequently causes no signs. You could begin to feel signs when a peripheral vein is no less than 60% hindered. A key sign is an irregular claudication. This is a leg cramp that fires up while you're moving around however at that point stops when you rest. It's an indication of decreased bloodstream brought about by the developing plaque in your artery. PAD can lead to significant issues in your legs and feet in addition to somewhere else in your body. That is because all your veins are associated with your cardiovascular framework. In this way, plaque development in one region dials back your entire organization of "pipes". PAD isn't equivalent to coronary artery disease (CAD), yet the two circumstances are connected. Individuals with one condition are probably going to have the other one, as well. Both PAD and CAD have a considerable lot of similar threat factors.

Hypertension

Hypertension and excessive cholesterol are connected. Cholesterol plaque and calcium make your supply routes hard and limited. Along these lines, your heart needs to strain a lot harder to transport blood through them. Accordingly, your circulatory strain turns out to be too high. High pulse and excessive cholesterol are two of the greatest reasons for coronary disease. In the U.S., around 1 out of 3 grown-ups have hypertension, and around 1 out of every 3 grown-ups have elevated cholesterol. For the greater part of the grown-ups in each gathering, treatment isn't helping enough or, more than likely they're not utilizing any treatment. Medications from your medical care supplier can help a lot, yet a way of life changes can assist those medication with working at their best. Way of life changes are significant for overseeing both excessive cholesterol and hypertension. A few changes include:

* Eat less immersed fat and trans fat: Quick food can contain high measures of both. Yet, even food sources at formal eateries can be high in immersed fat contingent upon how they're cooked.

* Eat less frizzled food and handled food varieties: These incorporate prepackaged pastries and bites.

* Eat less sodium (salt): A few food varieties have stowed away the salt. Perusing marks in the store is significant. A few cafés might have the option to share sustenance data for menu items.

* Quit smoking and utilizing tobacco items: Smoking is a main threat factor for coronary disease and vein issues.

What clinical issues influence my cholesterol levels

Clinical issues and cholesterol have a two-way relationship. Excessive cholesterol can lead to clinical issues like atherosclerosis. Be that as it may, a few ailments can likewise put you at a higher threat of having excessive cholesterol. Here are a few circumstances that might influence your cholesterol levels;

Chronic kidney disease (CKD): Individuals with Chronic kidney disease (CKD) face a higher threat of creating coronary artery disease. That is because CKD makes plaque develop all the more rapidly in their supply routes. Individuals with beginning phase CKD are debound to pass on from coronary disease rather than kidney disease. CKD makes you have more fatty oils (a sort of fat) in your blood. It likewise makes you have exceptionally low-density lipoprotein (VLDL) cholesterol. VLDLs are particles that carry fatty oil. In the interim, CKD brings down your "good cholesterol" (HDL) levels and keeps your HDLs from functioning as they ought to. CKD additionally changes the construction of your "Bad cholesterol" (LDL) particles so they hurt more.

HIV(human immunodeficiency Virus): Individuals with HIV are almost two times as possible as individuals without HIV to have a coronary failure or stroke. Analysts used to think this higher threat came from HIV meds (antiretroviral treatment). They accepted those prescriptions raised an individual's cholesterol. Yet, more current exploration shows the guilty party is an individual's insusceptible system. Even if your HIV is made due, your safe framework might in any case be enacted. This places your body in a condition of constant irritation. This irritation triggers plaque development and atherosclerosis. Fortunately, individuals with HIV are living longer. Yet, that implies more examination needs to investigate what ongoing chronic diseases like heart disease mean for them.

Thyroid illness: Having thyroid sickness can influence your cholesterol levels. That is because the thyroid chemical impacts how your body processes lipids (fats). The effect relies upon what sort of thyroid illness you have.

Hyperthyroidism: This condition makes your body make a lot of thyroid chemicals. Meds used to treat this condition can raise your cholesterol levels (aggregate, LDL, and HDL). Assuming you're being treated for hyperthyroidism, talk with your medical services supplier about how to deal with your cholesterol.

Hypothyroidism: This condition makes your body make too minimal thyroid chemicals. It additionally makes you have more excessive cholesterol levels. For this situation, treatment for thyroid sickness brings down your cholesterol levels. However, you might in any case have to take statins to get your cholesterol in the best reach

Lupus: Individuals with lupus as a rule have more significant levels of "bad cholesterol" (LDL, VLDL) and fatty oils. They likewise have lower levels of "good cholesterol" (HDL).

Individuals who have dynamic lupus face a more serious threat of Excessive cholesterol contrasted and the people who have very much made-due (calm) lupus. Lupus raises the possibility of creating coronary artery disease. That is in view of the fact that lupus puts your body in a condition of persistent irritation. This irritation prompts quicker plaque development in your arteries.

Polycystic ovary syndrome (PCOS): Individuals with polycystic ovary syndrome (PCOS) face a higher risk of coronary illness. This hazard goes up more as they age. PCOS raises the risk of numerous coronary illness risk factors, including diabetes and hypertension. Individuals with PCOS are bound to have high "bad cholesterol" (LDL) levels and low "good cholesterol" (HDL) levels.

Diabetes mellitus: Diabetes mellitus (Type 1 diabetes and Type 2 diabetes) copies your threat for coronary artery disease and peripheral artery disease. Diabetes is connected with lower levels of HDLs and more significant levels of fatty substances and LDLs.About 7 out of 10 individuals with Type 2 diabetes are determined to have diabetes-related dyslipidemia. This implies they have high fatty substance levels, high "Small dense" LDL levels, and low HDL levels. "Small dense" LDL is a particular kind of cholesterol protein that can undoubtedly enter your artery wall and cause harm. Having an excessive number of small dense LDLs in your blood can make plaque develop.

Chapter 2

Hurtful truth about vegetable oil

In opposition to mainstream thinking, the simple truth that vegetable oil is obtained from vegetables doesn't make it valuable to your well-being. Part of the fault for this is credited to the food organizations showcasing their items in manners that aren't guaranteed to uncover every bit of relevant information. Today, we investigate the confusing universe of vegetable oils to expose a few misinterpretations and lay out certain realities to help you in your well-being journey. Vegetable oils are palatable oils, reaped from a grouping of plants. Vegetable oils are capable of additives, improving the life span of food items. Despite the fact that they are habitually utilized in our culinary interests, for example, cooking and baking, it is through handled food sources like cheap food, bundled food varieties, salad dressings, and fixings that the majority of our vegetable oil utilization takes place. The creation and handling of vegetable oils is the thing we ought to address. The handling technique fundamentally decides if the oil actuates a provocative or calming reaction in our bodies. The test then lies in figuring out which oil variations are valuable to our wellbeing and which are not, so you can zero in on the right ones.

Tip No. 1: Settle on raw vegetable oils: Diving into the creation interaction of refined vegetable oils, we find that it generally includes a substance dissolvable to remove the oil from the plant. The resulting purging, refinement, and intermittent synthetic changes can deliver these oils unsatisfactory for a solid body. Refined oil examples include soybean oil, corn oil, canola, hydrogenated oils, and grapeseed oil. Conversely, crude vegetable oils obtained from plant or seed smashing or squeezing without utilizing hurtful synthetics, are better. This classification includes olive oil, avocado oil, grapeseed oil, and coconut oil. Curiously, grapeseed oil shows up on the two records, illustrating that there are crude adaptations of different oils.

Tip No. 2: Exercise attention with health affirmations of vegetable oils: While all vegetable oils convey the "heart healthy" tag ascribed to their polyunsaturated fat substance (which is healthier than soaked fat), this may not be the whole truth. Corn oil or soybean oil might seem better than immersed fats, for example: coconut oil, yet this perspective disregards the oil's plant beginning, handling strategies, and utilization amount. Try not to be off track by working on wellbeing claims. Refined corn oil and refined soybean oil, prevalently utilized in the food business, ought to in a perfect world be rejected from your eating regimen. Start examining your food bundle fixing records and note the recurrence of canola, corn, and soybean oil, which are all unhealthier choices.

Tip No. 3: Focus on perusing fixings records and pick better vegetable oils: Recognizing vegetable oils on fixing records is basically as critical as spotting refined sugar. What oil variation is in your "better" pack of chips or wafers? It's basic to be aware. The accompanying oils are all right with some restraint. Most contain excessive degrees of Omega-6 unsaturated fats, so they ought not to be consumed openly. In any case, they are viewed as normal fats and do have medical advantages. They are not perfect for high-intensity cooking, however adequate in dressings, mayos, and other non-heat foods. There are Pecan Oil, Flaxseed Oil, and Macadamia Nut Oil. Here is the large rundown I keep away from however much as could be expected. They are just not regular, and many are made with a comparable cycle to vegetable oil. Avoid these: Canola Oil, Corn Oil, Soybean Oil, Vegetable oil, Nut Oil, Sunflower Oil, Safflower Oil, Cottonseed Oil, Grapeseed Oil, Margarine, and Any phony spread substitutes. Essentially passing by these oils in the supermarket is easy. However, remember that most handled food varieties contain these oils, as well. Salad dressing, sauces, saltines, chips… actually look at your fixings. Try not to get them. Simply skip handled food sources and you'll save yourself a difficult situation. Exploring the intricate domain of vegetable oils requires informed direction. Try not to succumb to the distortion that all vegetable oils are solid. Focus on crude over refined oils, question well-being cases, and focus on fixing records on food bundles. Keep in mind, while advertising efforts could depict a few oils as better, actually more nuanced. Utilize these tips to settle on better decisions, and recall, with regards to vegetable oils, they genuinely aren't indistinguishable.

PART TWO

Living Long and Better

Chapter 3

Shedding Fat by Irregular Fasting

Irregular fasting refers to a diet schedule that cycles between not eating and eating. Patterns of irregular fasting can be hourly or every day. An individual might practice while fasting, yet safeguards are necessary. People might decide to fast because of reasons like religion, diet, or potential medical advantages. During irregular fasting (IF), individuals might wish to start working out.

Why individuals might exercise while fasting

Individuals who are fasting can participate in working out. Certain individuals practice IF as they accept it has potential medical advantages. These include:

Weight loss: When individuals eat starches, the body changes over this into a sort of sugar known as glucose. The body stores glucose as glycogen. During times of fasting, glycogen stores are vacant. This implies the body begins to consume fat for energy during exercise, which might assist with weighting misfortune. Practicing in an abstained state likewise prompted a higher fat misfortune than in individuals practicing after a meal. However, different examinations have delivered different results. To get fitter, the calories somebody consumes should be not exactly those they consume every day. I may assist an individual with getting fitter as it controls the number of calories they eat.

Autophagy: Autophagy is a cycle that obliterates undesirable or harmed cells to recover more current and better ones.

Anti-aging: IF and exercise might slow back maturing and infection processes. This is because IF and exercise might cause changes in metabolism.

Kinds of Irregular fasting

There are various kinds of irregular fasting. These include:

16:8; During 16:8 fasting, an individual won't eat anything for 16 hours and afterward have an 8-hour window where they devour food. During the 16 hours of fasting, individuals can drink non-calorie refreshments, like dark espresso, dark tea, and water.

5:2; The 5:2 eating routine is a sort of quick where an individual eats ordinarily for 5 days and dispenses 2 days of fasting.

Daily: Daily fasting includes having a drawn-out period, enduring from the night to the next morning, without food. A delayed fasting of 13 hours short-term might diminish the risk of bosom malignant growth in females.

Up-to-the-10th hour: During this fasting, an individual won't eat nourishment for the initial 8 hours of their waking day. From the ninth hour, the individual can then eat.

One feast a day (OMAD): OMAD fasting includes picking one dinner daily to eat and spending the remainder of the day fasting.

Alternate Day: As the name recommends, alternate day fasting is the point at which an individual eats food as typical one day and diets on the accompanying day. If individuals need to change their standard dietary patterns, it merits examining this with a specialist or nutritionist, particularly for a change like fasting.

Planning the exercise.

It means quite a bit to design exercises during IF to remain safe. A few contemplations are:

Kind of activity: There are two sorts of activity, oxygen-consuming and anaerobic. High-impact workout, or 'cardio,' is practice over a supported period, like running, strolling, and cycling. Anaerobic is a practice that requires the most extreme exertion over a brief period, for example, weight training or running. Which sort of activity an individual will probably rely upon the kind of fasting they do. For instance, an individual doing a 16:8 or daily diet can do either high-impact or anaerobic activity during their times of eating. However, to practice during their day of not eating, they ought to likely adhere to less extreme vigorous activity.

Timing of the activity: Although an individual can practice in an abstained state, timing exercise for after meals might be better.

Sort of food: On the off chance that practicing during times of eating, it is essential to consider what to eat. Pre-exercise sustenance ought to comprise a feast 2-3 hours before practice instead of not long previously. It very well may be wealthy in complex sugars, for example, entire grain cereal and protein. A post-exercise feast ought to comprise starches, top-notch proteins, and fats to help recuperation.

Safety Tips

After arranging the exercise, it is likewise worth thinking about the accompanying tips to remain safe:

Practicing after times of eating: This will furnish an individual with the energy they need to finish an exercise.

Adhering to low-force works out: If in an abstained express, an individual might wish to attempt to do power oxygen-consuming activity. Be that as it may, on the off chance that practicing after eating, doing any kind of exercise is generally protected.

Paying attention to what the body is talking about: If somebody is beginning to feel unwell during exercise while on IF, they ought to stop.

Remaining hydrated: In any event, when not On the off chance that, it is vital to keep hydrated during exercise. As the vast majority of the human body is water, it is imperative to supplant liquids lost during exercise.

For certain individuals fasting and practicing might be more dangerous, including Individuals with diabetes, Individuals with low circulatory strain, Individuals who have recently had scattered eating, Pregnant ladies, Ladies who are breastfeeding.

Chapter 4

Osteopenia,osteoporosis and   other bones issues

Osteopenia

Osteopenia is a deficiency of bone mineral density (BMD) that debilitates bones. It's more considered normal in individuals more seasoned than 50, particularly ladies. Osteopenia has no signs or side effects, however, an easy screening test can gauge bone strength. A certain way of life changes can assist you with safeguarding bone density and forestall osteoporosis.

What is osteopenia

Osteopenia is a deficiency of bone mineral density (BMD). Lower BMD demonstrates you have fewer minerals in your bones than you ought to, which makes bones more fragile

What causes osteopenia

Bones are made of living tissue. Up until about age 30, a sound individual forms more bone than the person in question loses. Yet, after age 35, bones start to separate quicker than they develop. Indeed, even in a solid individual, bone density diminishes throughout life, by under 1% each year. A few things can get bone misfortune going all the more rapidly, prompting osteopenia, for example,

* Ailments like hyperthyroidism.

* Drugs, for example, prednisone and a few therapies for malignant growth, indigestion, hypertension, and seizures.

* Hormonal changes during menopause.

* Unfortunate sustenance, particularly an eating regimen too low in calcium or vitamin D.

What are the signs of osteopenia

Osteopenia normally causes no signs or side effects until it advances to osteoporosis. Seldom, certain individuals with osteopenia may encounter bone torment or shortcomings. The condition is normally distinguished when an individual has a BMD screening.

How are osteopenic bones treated

There's no solution for osteopenia, yet saving bone density however much as could be expected is significant. Treatment includes basic techniques to keep your bones as sound areas of strength for conceivable and forestall movement to osteoporosis: Calcium treatment, working out, Solid eating routine, Supplements for lack of vitamin D, and openness to the sun to assist your body with retaining vitamin D.

What can I do to prevent bone loss

A few procedures can assist you with keeping up with bone strength and forestall bone misfortune:

* Abstain from smoking.

* Eat a solid, offset diet with heaps of natural products, vegetables, calcium, and nutrients.

* Work out each day; Strolling, running, and different exercises that make you bear your weight are especially useful, as is weight lifting.

* Get no less than 1,200 mg of calcium every day.

* Get somewhere around 800 to 1,000 IU of vitamin D day to day.

* Go outside for openness to the sun, which assists your body with engrossing vitamin D into the circulation system.

* Limit liquor.

O steoporosis

Osteoporosis is an infection that debilitates your bones. It makes your bones more slender and less dense than they ought to be. Individuals with osteoporosis are substantially more likely to encounter broken bones (bone fractures). Your bones are generally dense and sufficiently able to help your weight and retain most sorts of effects. As you age, your bones normally lose a portion of their thickness and their capacity to regrow (rebuild) themselves. On the off chance that you have osteoporosis, your bones are considerably more delicate than they ought to be and are a lot more fragile.

Many people don't realize they have osteoporosis until it makes them break a bone. Osteoporosis can make any of your bones bound to break, however, the most usually impacted bones include your; Hips (hip breaks), Wrists, and Spine (cracked vertebrae).

How normal is osteoporosis

More than 50 million individuals in the U.S. live with osteoporosis and it's normal in individuals over 50. Specialists gauge that portion surprisingly of all people assigned female at birth and 1 in 4 people assigned male at birth over 50 have osteoporosis. 1 of every 3 grown-ups more than 50 who don't have osteoporosis yet have some level of diminished bone density (osteopenia). Individuals with osteopenia have early indications of osteoporosis. If it's not treated, osteopenia can become osteoporosis.

What are osteoporosis signs

Osteoporosis doesn't have signs like bunches of other ailments do. That is the reason medical services suppliers at times consider it a quiet disease. You won't feel or notice whatever that signals you could have osteoporosis. You will not have a migraine, fever, or stomachache that tells you something in your body is off-base. The most well-known "sign" is unexpectedly breaking a bone, particularly after a little fall or minor accident that normally wouldn't hurt you. Even though osteoporosis doesn't straightforwardly cause signs, you could see a couple of changes in your body that can mean your bones are losing strength or density. These warning signs of osteoporosis can include Losing an inch or a greater amount of your level, Changes in your regular stance (stooping or bowing forward more), Shortness of breath (If the desk in your spine is adequately compacted to lessen your lung limit), Lower back torment (torment in your lumbar spine).

What causes osteoporosis

Osteoporosis occurs as you progress in years and your bones lose their capacity to regrow and change themselves. Your bones are living tissue like some other piece of your body. It probably won't seem like it, yet they're continually supplanting their cells and tissue all through your life. Up until about age 30, your body normally constructs more bone than you lose. After age 35, bone breakdown happens quicker than your body can supplant it, which causes a progressive deficiency of bone mass. If you have osteoporosis, you lose bone mass at a more prominent rate. Individuals in postmenopause lose bone mass considerably quicker.

How is osteoporosis treated

The most well-known osteoporosis medicines include:

Work out: Normal activity can reinforce your bones (and all the tissue associated with them, similar to your muscles, ligaments, and tendons). Your supplier could propose a weight-bearing activity to fortify your muscles and train your equilibrium. Practices that make your body neutralize gravity like strolling, yoga, Pilates, and kendo can work on your solidarity and equilibrium without putting a lot of weight on your bones. You could have to work with an actual specialist to find activities and developments that are ideal for you.

Nutrient and mineral enhancements: You could require over-the-counter or remedy calcium or vitamin D enhancements. Your supplier will let you know which type you want, how frequently you ought to take them, and which measurement you'll require.

Drugs for osteoporosis: Your supplier will let you know which solutions will turn out best for yourself as well as your body. Probably the most well-known drugs suppliers use to deal with osteoporosis incorporate chemical treatments like substitution estrogen or testosterone and bisphosphonates. Individuals with extreme osteoporosis or a high risk of breaks could require meds, including parathyroid chemical (PTH) analogs, denosumab, and romosozumab. These meds are normally given as injection

Prevention of osteoporosis

Exercise and ensuring you get sufficient calcium and vitamin D in your eating routine are normally everything you'll have to forestall osteoporosis. Your supplier will assist you with finding a mix of medicines that is best for yourself as well as your bone health. Follow these overall security tips to decrease your risks of a physical issue:

* Continuously wear your safety belt.

* Wear the right defensive hardware for movements of every kind and sport.

* Ensure your home and work area are liberated from the mess that could trip you or others.

* Continuously utilize the appropriate apparatuses or hardware at home to arrive at things. On no occasion should you stand on seats, tables, or ledges.

* Follow an eating regimen and exercise plan that is smart for you.

* Utilize a stick or walker if you experience issues strolling or have an expanded risk for falls.

PART THREE:Reverting ofDisease

C hapter 5

Greasy liver and Greasy kidney disease

Steatotic (Greasy) Liver disease

Steatotic liver disease (SLD) includes having an abundance of fat in your liver. Metabolic circumstances and weighty liquor use are risk factors. Contingent upon the sort of SLD you have, the fat development may not create issues, or it might prompt liver harm. Frequently, you can forestall or try and converse SLD with meds and way of life changes.

What is steatotic (greasy) liver disease

Steatotic liver disease (SLD) incorporates a few circumstances related to steatosis in your liver. "Steatosis" is a term medical care suppliers use to depict fat development in an organ (normally your liver). A solid, advanced liver contains a limited quantity of fat. Fat development turns into an issue when it comes to more than 5% of your liver's weight.

What are the kinds of steatotic (greasy) liver disease

Alcohol-related liver disease (ALD)
With ALD, steatosis happens given extreme alcohol utilization. Each time your liver channels alcohol a portion of its cells kick the bucket. Generally, your liver can make new cells to supplant the old ones, so there isn't an issue. Yet, if you drink an excess of alcohol your liver will most likely be unable to keep up. All things being equal, steatosis may set in.

Non-alcohol related liver disease (NAFLD)
Non-alcoholic liver disease (NAFLD) is the term for a scope of conditions brought about by the development of fat in the liver. Normally found in individuals who are overweight or corpulent. A sound liver should contain essentially no fat. With NAFLD, the guilty party has cardiometabolic risk factors. These variables incorporate circumstances and qualities that pose dangers to your heart health.

Risk factors related to NAFLD include Obesity, Type 2 diabetes, Hypertension, and Lipid irregularities (lipids are greasy mixtures tracked down in cells).

NAFLD applies assuming you polish off modest quantities of alcohol week by week. "Modest quantities" signifies under 140 grams each week for individuals assigned female at birth(AFAB) and under 210 grams each week for individuals assigned male at birth (AMAB). For reference, in the U.S., one norm, 12-oz. lager contains around 14 grams of liquor.

Metabolic-associated steatohepatitis (MASH)
Metabolic-associated steatohepatitis (MASH) is a serious type of NAFLD. With MASH, fat development advances to aggravation, then, at that point, tissue harm and scarring (fibrosis). Beforehand, medical care suppliers alluded to MASH as non-alcohol-related steatohepatitis (NASH).

NAFLD and increased alcohol intake (MetALD)
If you have MetALD, both metabolic risk elements and alcohol utilization assume a part in fat development in your liver. With MetALD, you have a cardiometabolic risk factor and polish off more than 140 grams each week (AFAB) or more than 210 grams each week (AMAB). What contributes most to the fat

development in your liver (alcohol utilization or metabolic risk factors) shifts from one individual to another.

Is steatotic (greasy) liver disease a difficult issue

By and large, the fat development doesn't create difficult issues or keep your liver from working normally. In a few cases, the condition advances to liver illness. It as a rule advances in stages:

Hepatitis: Your liver goes from greasy to kindled (enlarged). The irritation harms tissue. This stage is called steatohepatitis. For instance, this happens when NAFLD becomes a Pound.

Fibrosis: Groups of scar tissue structure where the aggravation harms your liver, making it harden. This interaction is called fibrosis.

Cirrhosis: Broad scar tissue replaces solid tissue. As of now, you have cirrhosis of the liver. Without therapy, cirrhosis can prompt possibly lethal circumstances like liver disappointment and liver disease. Around 90% of individuals who create hepatocellular carcinoma (HCC) — a kind of liver disease — have cirrhosis. This is the reason it's so essential to realize what's causing fat development in your liver and get treated. Regardless of whether you have beginning phase cirrhosis, there are steps you can take to shield your liver from additional harm. On certain occasions, you might turn around some harm by following your supplier's treatment plan for you.

What are the signs of steatotic (greasy) liver disease

SLD doesn't necessarily cause signs. At the point when they're available, signs include Stomach torment or a sensation of completion in the upper right half of your midsection (gut), Outrageous weariness or shortcoming (weakness). All the more normally, individuals notice side effects once SLD has advanced to cirrhosis of the liver. At the point when cirrhosis occurs, you might insight: Queasiness, Loss of craving, Unexplained weight reduction, Yellowish skin and whites of the eyes (jaundice), Enlarging in your mid-region (ascites), Expanding in your legs, feet, or hands (edema), Dying (that your supplier tracks down in your throat, stomach or rectum).

What causes steatotic (greasy) liver disease

SLD has various causes. In any case, you're bound to foster SLD if you have a cardiometabolic risk factor, if you drink undesirable measures of alcohol or both. You have a more prominent possibility of creating SLD if you:

* Have liquor use jumble (regular or weighty liquor use).

* Have metabolic disorders (insulin opposition, hypertension, elevated cholesterol, and high fatty oil levels).

* Have Type 2 diabetes.

* Have overweight (BMI 25 to 29.9 kilograms kg/m2).

* Have weight (BMI 30 kg/m2 or more).

* Have polycystic ovary disorder (PCOS).

* Have obstructive rest apnea.

* Have hypothyroidism (low thyroid chemicals).

* Have hypopituitarism (low pituitary organ chemicals).

* Have hypogonadism (low sex chemicals).

What are the difficulties of SLD

Without therapy, a steatotic liver can advance to cirrhosis of the liver, which can prompt liver disappointment, liver malignant growth, and diseases outside your liver. Individuals with MASLD are likewise at an expanded chance of coronary disease. Coronary disease — not liver disease — is the main source of death in individuals with NAFLD.

How is steatotic (greasy) liver disease treated

There's no particular treatment or prescription. All things considered, suppliers center around assisting you with overseeing risk factors that add to the condition. This includes making way of life changes that can work on your well-being. These are:

Keep away from alcohol: Avoid alcohol regardless of whether your SLD isn't connected with liquor use.

Shed pounds: Working out, changing what you eat and drink (under the oversight of a nutritionist), and taking meds, like GLP1RA, can assist with weight reduction. You might fit the bill for a bariatric medical procedure, which can likewise assist you with getting more fit.

Take drugs to oversee metabolic circumstances: Take recommended meds to oversee diabetes, cholesterol, and fatty substances (fat in the blood). You may likewise have to take vitamin E and thiazolidinediones (drugs used to treat diabetes, like Actos® and Avandia®) in unambiguous cases.

Receive an immunization shot for hepatitis A and hepatitis B: These viral contaminations are particularly perilous if you as of now have liver illness.

Fatty Kidney Disease

Fatty kidney disease is the impact of renal ectopic fat adding to persistent kidney disease. Persistent kidney disease is the diminished capacity of the kidney to do these capabilities in the long haul. This is most frequently brought about by harm to the kidneys from different circumstances, most normally diabetes and hypertension.

What does your kidney do

The kidneys are 2 bean-molded organs, the size of your clenched hand. They're situated on one or the other side of the body, just underneath the ribcage. The principal job of the kidneys is to channel byproducts from the blood before changing them into pee. The kidneys moreover:

* Assist with keeping up with circulatory strain

* Keep up with the right degrees of synthetic compounds in your body, thus, will assist the heart and muscles with working appropriately

* Produce the dynamic type of vitamin D that keeps bones solid

* Produce a substance called erythropoietin, which invigorates creation of red platelets

What are the 5 phases of chronic kidney Disease

There are five phases of chronic kidney disease. The stages depend on how well your kidneys can sift through squander from your blood. Blood and pee tests figure out which phase of CKD you're in.

Stage I: Slight harm to the kidney(s) harm

Stage II: Gentle decline in kidney capability

Stage III: Moderate reduction in kidney capability

Stage IV: Serious abatement in kidney capability

Stage V: Kidney disappointment

What are the signs of chronic kidney disease

In the beginning phases of kidney disease you for the most part don't have observable side effects. As the infection declines, signs might include A need to pee more regularly, Sluggishness, shortcomings, low energy level, Loss of hunger, Expanding of your hands, feet and lower legs, Windedness, Frothy or effervescent pee, Puffy eyes, Dry and irritated skin, Inconvenience concentrating, Inconvenience resting, Deadness, Queasiness or heaving, Muscle cramps, Hypertension, Obscuring of your skin. Remember that it can require a long time for waste to develop in your blood and cause signs

What are the normal causes of kidney disease

Hypertension (hypertension) and diabetes are the two most normal reasons for constant kidney disease. Different causes and conditions that influence kidney capability and can cause constant kidney disease include

Glomerulonephritis: This sort of kidney disease includes harm to the glomeruli, which are the filtering units inside your kidneys.

Polycystic kidney disease: This is a hereditary problem that makes numerous liquid-filled pimples fill in your kidneys, decreasing the capacity of your kidneys to work.

Membranous nephropathy: Here your body's resistant framework goes after the waste-filtering layers in your kidney.

Vesicoureteral reflux: This is a condition wherein pee streams in reverse back up your ureters to your kidneys.

Nephrotic condition: This is an assortment of signs that demonstrate kidney harm.

Diabetes-related nephropathy: This is harm or brokenness of at least one nerve, brought about by diabetes.

Lupus and other insusceptible framework illnesses that cause kidney issues; including polyarteritis nodosa, sarcoidosis, Goodpasture disorder, and Henoch-Schönlein purpura.

Who is in danger of chronic kidney disease

Anybody can get chronic kidney disease. You're more in danger of ongoing kidney sickness if you:

* Have diabetes.

* Have hypertension.

* Have coronary illness.

* Have a family background of kidney illness.

* Have strange kidney construction or size.

* Are over 60 years of age.

* Have a long history of taking NSAID (nonsteroidal anti-inflammatory drugs) painkillers. This includes over-the-counter (OTC) items and some solution painkillers.

How is chronic kidney disease treated

There's no remedy for constant kidney disease (CKD), however, steps can be taken to save your kidney capability so they fill into the extent that this would be possible. Assuming you have diminished kidney capability:

* Make and keep your customary medical care supplier/nephrologist (kidney-trained professional) visits. These suppliers screen your kidney's wellbeing.

* Deal with your blood glucose (sugar) if you have diabetes.

* Try not to take pain relievers and different prescriptions that might worsen your kidney.

* Deal with your pulse levels.

* Follow a kidney-accommodating eating routine.Dietary changes might incorporate restricting protein, eating food sources that diminish blood cholesterol levels, and restricting sodium (salt) and potassium consumption.

* Try not to smoke.

* Work out/be dynamic on most days of the week.

* Remain at a weight that is smart for you.

Forestalling persistent kidney disease

The fundamental method for decreasing the possibilities of CKD creation is to guarantee any current circumstances, for example, diabetes and hypertension, are painstakingly made due. A few different things you can do to forestall CKD are:

* Deal with your hypertension.

* Manage your glucose expecting you to have diabetes.

* Eat an even eating routine.

* Try not to smoke or utilize tobacco.

* Be dynamic for 30 minutes no less than five days per week.

* Keep a sound weight.

* Take non-prescription painkillers just as coordinated. Taking more than coordinated can harm your kidneys.

* Limit liquor containing refreshments.

What food varieties are bad for kidneys

In individuals with solid kidneys, there aren't genuinely horrendous food varieties or food sources that hurt your kidneys. However, if you have CKD, your medical services supplier might suggest a kidney-accommodating eating routine. Components of a kidney-accommodating eating regimen might include:

* Staying away from food sources that are high in salt.This additionally assists control of blood pressure.

* Eating the perfect proportion of protein. Protein makes more waste than other nutrition types. In this way, since your kidneys eliminate squandering, bringing down protein can assist with protecting their capability.

* Eating heart-good food varieties.

* Eating food sources low in phosphorus. This incorporates new leafy foods and entire grains. Food sources like dairy and beans are high in phosphorus.

* Keep away from food varieties high in potassium like bananas, oranges, and potatoes.

PART FOUR: Living Great

Chapter 6

Frequent vitamins, Minerals and Nutrients disease

Vitamin deficiencies disease

Vitamin is a micronutrient that isn't ready by the body in adequate sums. This is the motivation behind why it is important to take in from outside hotspots for the ordinary working of the body. Deficient absorption of lack of nutrients brings about nutrient sicknesses. Following is the rundown of a portion of the nutrients and the deficiencies disease brought about by them:

Vitamin A

A significant micronutrient is obtained from various food sources like carrots, spinach, milk, egg, liver, and fish. It is expected for the typical vision, multiplication, development, and sound-resistant arrangement of an individual. Most youngsters under five years old experience the ill effects of xerophthalmia, a serious eye problem, in which the kid is in danger of becoming visually impaired. Lack of vitamin A in a pregnant lady can prompt entanglements during pregnancy and labor.

Vitamin B

Vitamin B can be of various sorts, for example, Vitamin B1, B2, B12 and so on. The deficiencies disease rely upon the sort of Vitamin B that an individual is lacking

Vitamin B1: Lack of vitamin B1 causes beriberi, which brings about frail muscles and extreme weight reduction. Intense inadequacy can prompt loss of motion and cardiovascular disappointment.

Vitamin B6: The absence of lack of vitamin B6 causes sicknesses, for example, anemia and certain skin problems like breaks around the mouth. It can likewise prompt wretchedness and mental meltdowns.

Vitamin B12: The absence of vitamin B12 causes malignant anemia. Different diseases connected with B12 lack are muscle and nerve loss of motion, outrageous weariness, dementia, and despondency.

Vitamin C

Lack of vitamin C can cause scurvy, an illness that is portrayed by draining gums, skin spots, and expanding in joints. It likewise influences the safe framework and could be deadly in intense circumstances.

Vitamin D

Lack of vitamin D causes rickets, which prompts the debilitating of bones, particularly close to the joints. It can likewise prompt the rot of teeth.

Vitamin K

Vitamin K is significant for blood coagulation. Its lack is normal in babies and prompts unreasonable draining because of the powerlessness to frame blood clusters.

Minerals deficiencies disease

Minerals are inorganic supplements that incorporate minor components like copper, zinc, iodine, and iron, alongside the micronutrients, for example, calcium, potassium, magnesium, and sodium. Following is the rundown of a couple of lack of minerals alongside the infections related to them:

Iodine

Iodine is the main component expected for the mental health of the fetus. It is liable for various capabilities like the creation of chemicals. Salt is a huge wellspring of iodine in various countries. The lack of iodine prompts goiter disease

Iron

Iron, as hemoglobin, conveys oxygen from the lungs to various tissues of the body. Lack of iron causes anaemia, a condition in which the blood can't convey the expected oxygen to the tissues, which likewise brings about death. Around 40-60% of newborn children in emerging nations experience the ill effects of mental weakness because of a lack of iron. Red meat, spinach, poultry, and so forth are a portion of the iron-rich food sources.

Nutritional diseases

Nutritional diseases are any of the supplement-related diseases and conditions that cause sickness in people. They might remember the lack of abundance for the eating regimen, stoutness, and dietary issues, and persistent sicknesses like cardiovascular disease, hypertension, malignant growth, and diabetes mellitus. Nutritional diseases likewise include formative anomalies that can be forestalled by diet, genetic metabolic problems that answer dietary therapy, the communication of food varieties and supplements with drugs, food sensitivities and prejudices, and possible perils in the food supply. Nutritional lacks are:

Dietary disease : Dietary disease is any of the supplement-related sicknesses and conditions that cause ailments in people. They might remember a lack or surplus for the eating routine, corpulence and dietary issues, and ongoing diseases like cardiovascular disease, hypertension, disease, and diabetes mellitus. Dietary disease likewise includes formative anomalies that can be forestalled by diet, genetic metabolic issues that answer dietary therapy, the communication of food varieties and supplements with drugs, food sensitivities and bigotries, and expected perils in the food supply.

Iodine: Iodine lack is a condition in which iodine is deficient or isn't used as expected. Iodine is a component that straightforwardly influences thyroid organ emissions, which themselves by and large control heart activity, nerve reaction to boosts, pace of body development, and digestion.

Dehydration : Dehydration, and loss of water from the body; it is constantly connected with some deficiency of salt (sodium chloride). The treatment of any type of lack of hydration, in this manner, requires not just the substitution of the water lost from the body yet also the reclamation of the typical convergence of salt inside the body fluid. This assists with supplanting water lost from the body, as well as reestablishing salt focuses to typical levels inside body fluids. Dehydration might be brought about by confined water consumption, extreme water misfortune, or both. The most well-known reason for lack of hydration is the inability to drink fluids. The hardship of water is undeniably more serious than the hardship of food. The typical individual loses around 2.5 percent of absolute body water each day (around 1,200 milliliters [1.25 quarts]) in pee, in lapsed air, by torpid sweat, and from the gastrointestinal tract.

Obesity : Obesity is, an inordinate collection of muscle versus fat, typically brought about by the utilization of additional calories than the body can utilize. The abundance of calories is then put away as fat, or fat tissue. Overweight, if moderate, isn't obesity, especially in strong or huge-boned people.

Scurvy: Scurvy, one of the most established known nutritional disorders of humanity, is brought about by a dietary absence of Vitamin C(ascorbic acid), a supplement found in many new foods grown from the ground, especially citrus organic products. Vitamin C is significant in the development of collagen (a component of typical tissues), and any lack of the nutrient disrupts the ordinary tissue blend, an issue that underlies the clinical signs of the disorder. Symptoms of scurvy normally become evident in no less than a while of Vitamin C being missing from the eating regimen, by which time waiting pools of Vitamin C in fat, muscle, and different tissues have been drained. Introductory side effects of scurvy include exhaustion irritation and solidness of the joints and lower furthest points. As the condition advances, the gums grow and drain, and teeth might be released. Bleeding under the skin and in profound tissues, slow wound healing, anemia, and changes in character are different signs of advanced disease. Left untreated, death ensues, commonly because of bleeding or complications from disease.

Prevention of Inadequacy disease

The inadequacy disease can be forestalled in the following way:

* Eating basic, healthy food like groundnuts, soybeans, pulses, and so forth.

* Prolonged cooking and half-cooked food lose their dietary benefit. Saving cut vegetables and natural products for a more drawn-out period likewise obliterates their dietary benefit. Keeping away from this can forestall inadequacy disease

* Maturation and growth hold and increment the healthy benefits of food.

Chapter 7

What is Niacin (Vitamin B3)

Niacin is one of the eight B nutrients, and it's additionally called nutrient B3. There are two primary synthetic types of niacin: Nicotinic acid and niacinamide (now and again called nicotinamide). The two structures are found in food varieties as well as supplements. The key job of niacin in your body is to orchestrate the coenzymes nicotinamide adenine dinucleotide (NAD) and nicotinamide adenine dinucleotide phosphate (NADP), which are engaged with over 400 biochemical responses in your body — essentially connected with acquiring energy from the food you eat. Niacin is water-dissolvable, so your body doesn't store it. This additionally implies that your body can discharge abundance measures of the nutrient through pee if they are not required. Your body helps niacin through food, however, it additionally makes modest quantities from the amino acid tryptophan, which can be found in protein sources like turkey and other creature foods.Niacin is one of 8 sorts of B nutrients significant for all aspects of your body. You can obtain them from meat, fish, and nuts. Supplements are now and again a choice, yet you ought to counsel your primary care physician first.Niacin, otherwise called vitamin B3, is a significant supplement. All aspects of your body need it to work properly. As an enhancement, niacin might assist with bringing down cholesterol, ease joint inflammation, and lift cerebrum capability, among other benefits. However, it can likewise cause serious incidental effects if you take huge doses. As with all B nutrients, niacin helps convert food into energy by supporting compounds. Niacin is a significant part of NAD and NADP, two coenzymes engaged with cell digestion. It assumes a part in cell flagging and making and fixing DNA, as well as going about as a cell reinforcement.

Signs of Niacin (Vitamin B3)

These are a portion of the side effects of niacin lack: Skin rash or staining, dazzling red tongue, vomiting, constipation or loose bowels, sorrow, weakness, migraine, cognitive decline, loss of hunger.

Five(5) medical advantages of Niacin (B3)

1. Further development of blood fat levels

Niacin might assist with further developing your blood fat levels by expanding your HDL (good) cholesterol, lessening your LDL (bad) LDL cholesterol, and diminishing your fatty oil levels. This might mean a decline in coronary disease risk, although a few examinations have found no connection between niacin supplementation and a reduction in coronary disease risk or deaths. It likewise takes high portions of niacin, regularly 1,500 mg or more prominent, to accomplish blood fat level upgrades, which builds the risk of encountering upsetting or possibly unsafe side effects. For these reasons, niacin is certainly not an essential treatment for excessive cholesterol. It's essentially used to assist with further developing blood fat levels in individuals who can't endure statin drugs.

2. May reduce blood pressure

One job of niacin is to deliver prostaglandins, or synthetic compounds that assist your veins with enlarging — further developing the bloodstream and lessening circulatory strain. Consequently, niacin might assume a part in the counteraction or treatment of hypertension.

3. May assist with treating type 1 diabetes

Type 1 diabetes is an immune system sickness wherein your body assaults and obliterates insulin-making cells in your pancreas. Niacin can assist with safeguarding those cells and conceivably even lower the threat of type 1 diabetes in youngsters who have a higher possibility of fostering this condition. However, for individuals with type 2 diabetes, the job of niacin is more convoluted. On one hand, it can assist with bringing down the excessive cholesterol levels that are in many cases found in individuals with type 2 diabetes. On the other, it can increase glucose levels. Thus, individuals with diabetes who take niacin to treat excessive cholesterol additionally need to screen their glucose cautiously

4. Boost brain function

Your mind needs niacin — as a piece of the coenzymes NAD and NADP — to get energy and capability properly. In truth, cerebrum haze and, surprisingly, mental side effects are related to niacin deficiency. Some sorts of schizophrenia can be treated with niacin, as it fixes harm to synapses that are brought about by a lack of niacin. It could likewise assist with keeping the cerebrum solid in instances of Alzheimer's disease

5. Further develops skin wellbeing

Niacin shields skin cells from sun harm, whether it's utilized orally or applied as a lotion. It might assist with forestalling specific kinds of skin malignant growth too. One top-notch concentrate in more than 300 individuals at high risk of skin disease tracked down that taking 500 mg of nicotinamide two times every day decreased paces of nonmelanoma skin malignant growth contrasted with control.

Conclusion

Considering the huge number of individuals who are worried about their eating regimens and make endeavors to change their dietary examples, we infer that it is significant to acquire a superior comprehension of both the programmed and natural impacts that are liable for individuals not following up on their sincere goals for diet change.

The clarifications in this book uncover the underlying driver of illnesses, upon the disposal of which their appearances will vanish regardless of how extraordinary our openness to their realized causes might be.